KETO

FOR BEGINNERS

50 Delicious Recipes

to Get Healthy and Look Great

AURORA MARIE QUEEN

TABLE OF CONTENTS

BREAKFAST

1 - Vegetable Omelet Colorful

Preparation	Cooking	Servings
12 min	**8 min**	**6**

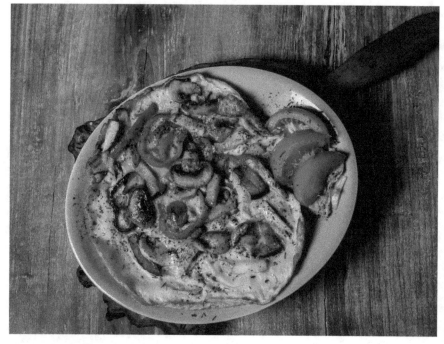

Ingredients

- 3 tablespoons olive oil
- 2 cup Chanterelle mushrooms, chopped
- 3 bell peppers, chopped
- 2 white onion, chopped
- 6 eggs

Direction

1. Heat the olive oil in a nonstick skillet over moderate heat. Now, cook the mushrooms, peppers, and onion until they have softened.

2. In a mixing bowl, whisk the eggs until frothy. Add the eggs to the skillet, reduce the heat to medium-low, and cook for approximately 5 minutes until the center starts to look dry. Do not overcook.

3. Taste and season with salt to taste.

Per Serving Calories: 237.2 Fat: 5.6g Carbohydrates: 10.1g Protein: 2.2g

2 - Fried Eggs

Preparation	Cooking	Servings
10 min	8 min	6

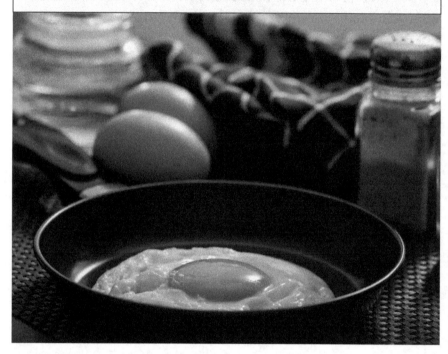

Ingredients

- 6 eggs
- 4 tbsp unsalted butter
- Seasoning:
- 1/2 tsp salt
- 1/4 tsp ground black pepper

Direction

1. Take a skillet pan, place it over medium heat, add butter and when it has melted, crack eggs in the pan.
2. Cook eggs for 3 to 5 minutes until fried to the desired level, then transfer the eggs to serving plates and sprinkle with salt and black pepper.
3. Serve.

Per Serving Calories: 19 Fat: 15 Carbohydrates: 0.8 Protein: 8.2g

3 - Beef and Egg Muffin

Preparation	Cooking	Servings
12 min	16 min	8

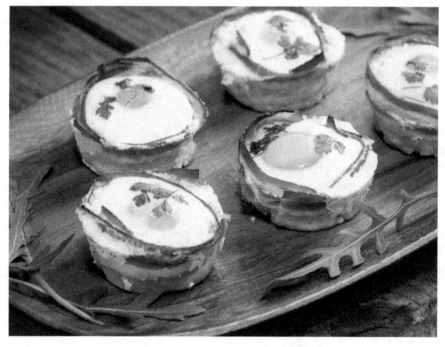

Ingredients

- 2 lbs of ground beef (20% fat/80% lean meat ratio)
- 1 tbsp of mixed herbs
- 8 eggs
- 1 cup of shredded cheddar cheese
- 2 cups of spinach

Direction

1. In a deep pan, saute the spinach with some olive oil for a few minutes until wilted. Remove from the heat and set aside.
2. In a 12-piece muffin, a tin dish begins lining each tin with around 1-2 tbsp of the ground beef to make a base cup. You should cover all sides of the tin and leave room for the spinach and eggs.
3. Top each meat cup with spinach, cheese, and one egg on top.
4. Cook in the oven for 15-18 minutes at 400F/200C

Per Serving: Calories: 224Fat: 17gCarbohydrates: 1.4gProtein: 15.7g

4 - Spicy Chili Eggs

Preparation	Cooking	Servings
15 min	45 min	6

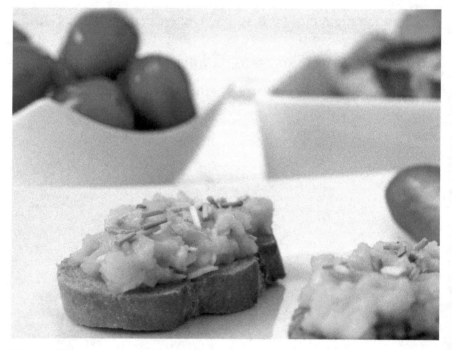

Ingredients

- 1/2 of lime, juiced
- 4 eggs, boiled
- 3 tsp chili garlic sauce
- 1 tsp paprika
- 1/4 tsp ground black pepper

Direction

1. Peel the boiled eggs, then slice in half lengthwise and transfer egg yolks to a medium bowl by using a spoon.
2. Mash the egg yolk, add remaining ingredients and stir until well combined.
3. Spoon the egg yolk mixture into egg whites and then serve.

Per Serving: Calories: 84Fat: 5.2gCarbohydrates: 0.5gProtein: 7.3g

5 - Egg Porridge

Preparation	Cooking	Servings
12 min	**15 min**	**6**

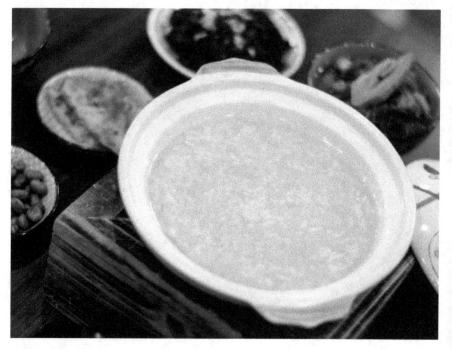

Ingredients

- 3 organic free-range eggs
- 1 / 2 cup organic heavy cream without food additives
- 3 packages of your preferred sweetener
- 3 tbsp grass-fed butter ground organic cinnamon to taste

Direction

1. In a bowl, add the eggs, cream, and sweetener, and mix together.
2. Melt the butter in a saucepan over medium heat. Lower the heat once the butter is melted.
3. Combine together with the egg and cream mixture.
4. While Cooking, mix until it thickens and curdles.
5. When you see the first signs of curdling, remove the saucepan immediately from the heat.
6. Pour the porridge into a bowl. Sprinkle cinnamon on top and serve immediately.

Per Serving: Calories: 565 Fat: 48g Carbohydrates: 2.3g Protein: 8.4g

APPETIZERS AND SNACKS

6 – Gluten Free Gratin

Preparation	Cooking	Servings
15 min	**22 min**	**6**

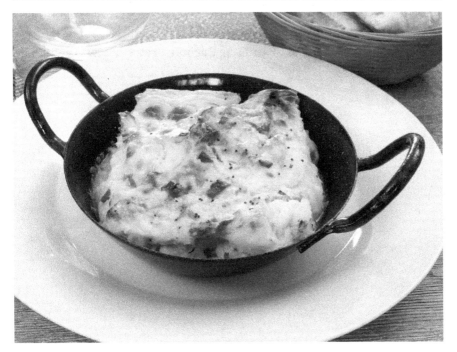

Ingredients

- 6 cups raw cauliflower florets
- 6 tbsp butter
- 1 / 2 cup heavy whipping cream
- Salt and pepper to taste
- 6 deli slices pepper jack cheese

Direction

1. Combine the cauliflower, butter, cream, salt, and pepper and microwave on medium for 20 minutes, or until tender.
2. Mash with a fork—season to your liking.
3. Lay the slices of cheese across the top of the cauliflower.
4. Cook inside your microwave for an additional 3 minutes, depending on the power of your microwave.
5. Serve!

Per Serving: Calories: 165 Fat: 14.3g Carbohydrates: 2.2g Protein: 4.2g

7 - Butternut Squash Cheese Bacon

Preparation	Cooking	Servings
15 min	**28 min**	**6**

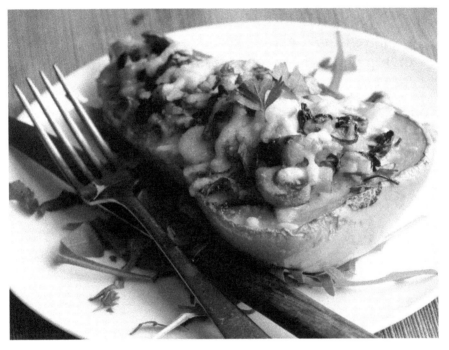

Ingredients

- 2 tablespoon olive oil
- 2 pound sliced butternut squash
- Kosher salt & Black pepper
- 2 cup grated Parmesan cheese
- 3 oz. chopped bacon

Direction

1. Set the oven to 4250F to preheat, then grease the baking tray
2. Add the olive oil in a medium skillet to heat to sauté the bacon, butternut squash, and the seasonings for 2 minutes.
3. After 2 minutes, pour everything on the baking tray to bake for 25 minutes
4. Remove from the oven, sprinkle the parmesan cheese on top the bake for 10 more minutes
5. Serve the meal while still warm.

Per Serving: Calories: 325 Fat: 32.3g Carbohydrates: 11.4g Protein: 24g

8 - Hot Buffalo Chicken Wings

Preparation	Cooking	Servings
20 min	4 hours	6

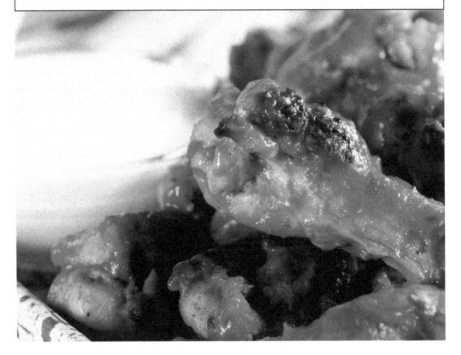

Ingredients

- 1 bottle of (12 ounces) hot pepper sauce
- 1 cup melted ghee
- 2 tablespoon dried oregano + onion powder
- 2 teaspoons garlic powder
- 4 pounds chicken wing sections

Direction

1. Take a large bowl and mix in hot sauce, ghee, garlic powder, oregano, onion powder, and mix well
2. Add chicken wings and toss to coat
3. Pour mix into Slow Cooker and cook on Low for 6 hours
4. Serve and enjoy!
Tip: If you don't have a slow cooker, you may use an Iron-Cast Dutch Oven. The temperature is 200 Degrees F for Low and 250 degrees F for High

Per Serving: Calories: 549 Fat: 3.2g Carbohydrates: 1.4g Protein: 30.3g

9 - Vanilla Pecans

Preparation	Cooking	Servings
15 min	2 hours	8

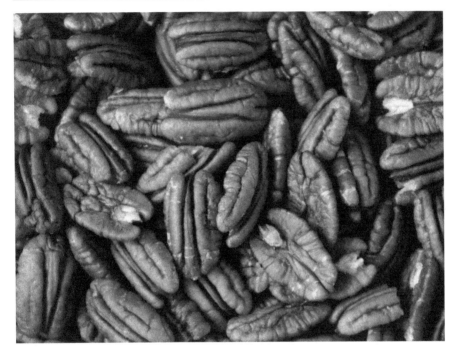

Ingredients

- 6 cups of raw pecans
- 1/2 cup of date paste
- 4 teaspoon of vanilla beans extract
- 2 teaspoon of sea salt
- 2 tablespoon of coconut oil

Direction

1. Add all of the listed ingredients to your pot

2. Cook on LOW for about 3 hours, making sure to stir it from time to time

3. Once done, allow it to cool and serve!

Per Serving: Calories: 345 Fat: 25g Carbohydrates: 15.2g Protein: 3.2g

10 - The Spaghetti Squash

Preparation	Cooking	Servings
10 min	**7 hours**	**8**

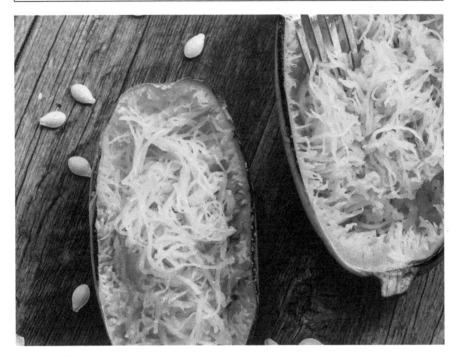

Ingredients

- 2 spaghetti squash
- 4 cups water

Direction

1. Wash squash carefully with water and rinse it well
2. Puncture 5-6 holes in the squash using a fork
3. Place squash in Slow Cooker
4. Place lid and cook on LOW for 7-8 hours

5. Remove squash to a cutting board and let it cool

6. Cut squash in half and discard seeds

7. Use two forks and scrape out squash strands and transfer to the bowl

8. Serve and enjoy!

Tip: If you don't have a slow cooker, you may use an Iron-Cast Dutch Oven. The temperature is 200 Degrees F for LOW and 250 degrees F for HIGH

Per Serving: Calories: 40 Fat: 50g Carbohydrates: 12.2g Protein: 1.3g

11 - Drumsticks Wrapped Bacon

Preparation	Cooking	Servings
15 min	**8 hours**	**8**

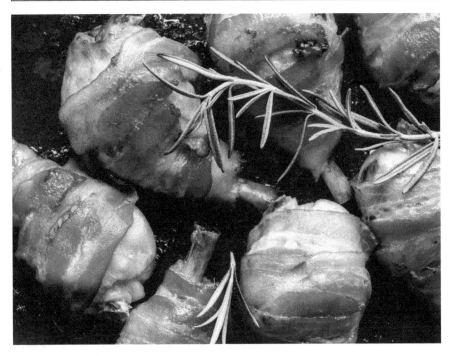

Ingredients

- 16 chicken drumsticks
- 16 slices thin-cut bacon

Direction

1. Wrap each chicken drumsticks in bacon
2. Place drumsticks in your Slow Cooker
3. Place lid and cook on Low for 8 hours
4. Serve and enjoy!

Tip: If you don't have a slow cooker, you may use an Iron-Cast Dutch Oven. The temperature is 200 Degrees F for Low and 250 degrees F for High

Per Serving: Calories: 212 Fat: 7g Carbohydrates: 3.2g Protein: 34g

12 - Cookie Coco Choco

Preparation	Cooking	Servings
15 min	0 min	8

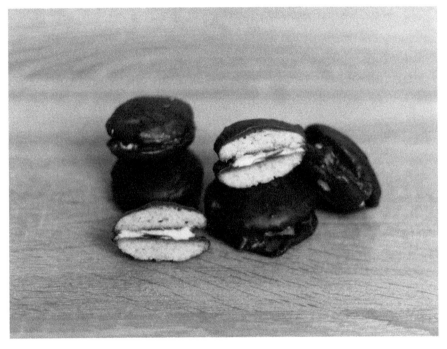

Ingredients

- 4 cups unsweetened coconut, shredded

- ½ cup coconut milk

- ¼ cup sugar-free maple syrup

- ¼ teaspoon almond extract

Direction

1. Blend coconut in your food processor until you have a nice texture.

2. Add coconut milk and syrup; keep blending until you have a nice batter.

3. Add more milk if the batter is a bit too crumbly.

4. Transfer the mixture to the mixing bowl.

5. Use your hand to form small balls.

6. Line a baking tray with parchment paper and transfer the balls, flatten them lightly to form a cookie shape.

7. Sprinkle coconut on top and chill for 2-3 hour until firm

8. Enjoy!

Per Serving: Calories: 47 Fat: 4.3g Carbohydrates: 3g Protein: 1.2g

BEEF

13 - Beef Bourguignon

Preparation	Cooking	Servings
15 min	60 min	6

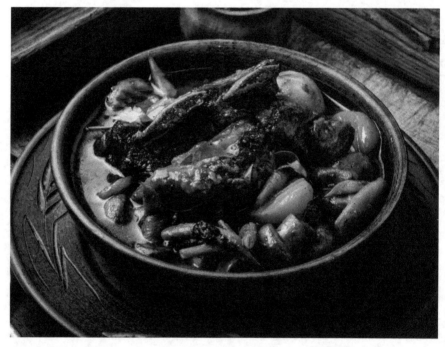

Ingredients

- 2 pounds shoulder steak, cut into cubes
- 2 tablespoon Herbs de Provence
- 2 onion, chopped
- 2 celery stalk, chopped
- 2 cup red Burgundy wine

Direction

1. Heat up a lightly greased soup pot over a medium-high flame. Now brown the beef in batches until no longer pink.
2. Add a splash of wine to deglaze your pan.
3. Add the Herbs de Provence, onion, celery, and wine to the pot; pour in 3 cups of water and stir to combine well. Bring to a rapid boil; then, turn the heat to medium-low.
4. Cover and let it simmer for 1 hour 10 minutes. Serve over hot cauliflower rice if desired. Enjoy!

Per Serving: Calories: 227 Fat: 4.2g Carbohydrates: 4.1g Protein: 22g

14 - Beef Mugs Cheddar and Zucchini

Preparation	Cooking	Servings
15 min	7 min	6

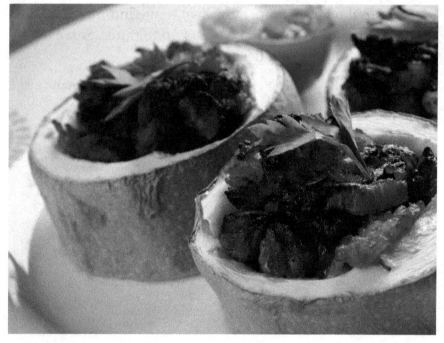

Ingredients

- 6 oz roast beef deli slices, torn apart
- 4 tbsp sour cream
- 2 small zucchini, chopped
- 3 tbsp chopped green chilies
- 4 oz shredded cheddar cheese

Direction

1. Divide the beef slices at the bottom of 2 wide mugs and spread 1 tbsp of sour cream.
2. Top with 2 zucchini slices, season with salt and pepper, add green chilies, top with the remaining sour cream, and then cheddar cheese.
3. Place the mugs in the microwave for 1-2 minutes until the cheese melts.
4. Remove the mugs, let cool for 1 minute, and serve.

Per Serving: Calories: 178 Fat: 9.2g Carbohydrates: 4.3g Protein: 17.1g

15 – Delicious Beef Stuffed Peppers

Preparation	Cooking	Servings
15 min	**45 min**	**6**

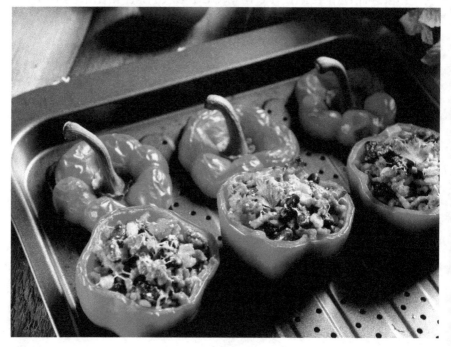

Ingredients

- 1 pound ground beef
- 2 garlic clove, minced
- Sea salt and ground black pepper, to taste
- 1/2 cup cream of onion soup
- 1 teaspoon paprika

Direction

1. Heat the olive oil in a saute pan over moderate heat. Once hot, sear the ground beef for 5 to 6 minutes, turning once or twice to ensure even cooking.
2. Add in the cream of onion soup, paprika, salt, and black pepper. Cook for a further 3 minutes until heated through. The meat thermometer should register 145 degrees F.
3. Serve in individual plates garnished with freshly snipped chives if desired. Enjoy!

Per Serving: Calories: 385 Fat: 24g Carbohydrates: 0.8g Protein: 41g

PORK

16 - Slow Cooked Pork Roast with Cranberry

Preparation	Cooking	Servings
15 min	9 hours	8

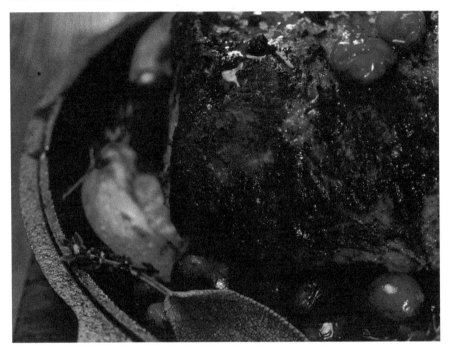

Ingredients

- 2 tablespoon coconut flour
- Salt and pepper to taste
- 3 pound pork loin
- Pinch of dry mustard
- 2 teaspoon ginger
- 4 tablespoons stevia
- 1 cup cranberries
- 4 garlic cloves, peeled and minced

- 1 lemon, sliced
- 1/2 cup water

Direction

1. Take a owl and add ginger, mustard, pepper and flour
2. Stir well
3. Add roast and toss well to coat it
4. Transfer meat to a Slow Cooker and add stevia, cranberries, garlic, water, lemon slices
5. Place lid and cook on LOW for 8 hours
6. Drizzle the pan juice on top and serve!

Per Serving: Calories: 440 Fat: 22g Carbohydrates: 3.2g Protein: 35g

17 - Spicy Pork Chops

Preparation	Cooking	Servings
4 hours	**20 min**	**6**

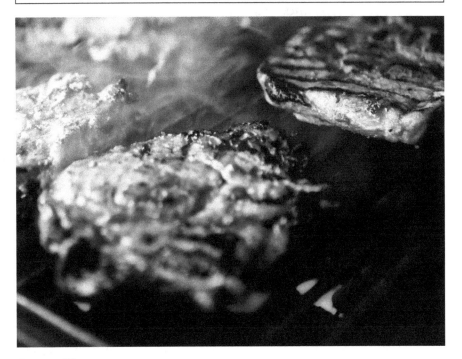

Ingredients

- 1/2 cup lime juice
- 6 pork rib chops
- 2 tablespoon coconut oil, melted
- 3 garlic cloves, peeled and minced
- 2 tablespoon chili powder
- 1 teaspoon ground cinnamon
- 3 teaspoons cumin
- Salt and pepper to taste

- 1 teaspoon hot pepper sauce
- Mango, sliced

Direction

1. Take a bowl and mix in lime juice, oil, garlic, cumin, cinnamon, chili powder, salt, pepper, hot pepper sauce
2. Whisk well
3. Add pork chops and toss
4. Keep it on the side and let it refrigerate for 4 hours
5. Pre-heat your grill to medium and transfer pork chops to pre-heated grill
6. Grill for 7 minutes, flip and cook for 7 minutes more
7. Divide between serving platters and serve with mango slices
8. Enjoy!

Per Serving: Calories: 210 Fat: 8.2g Carbohydrates: 3.1g Protein: 24g

POULTRY

18 - Chicken Lettuce Wraps

Preparation	Cooking	Servings
15 min	0 min	6

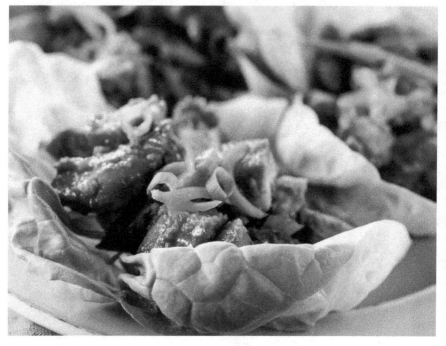

Ingredients

- 10 oz. of cooked chicken bites (roasted or boiled)
- 6 slices of fried beef bacon, chopped
- 1 cup of mayonnaise
- 6 large romaine lettuce leaves
- 2 large tomato seeded and cubed

Direction

1. Combine all the ingredients together except the lettuce leaves in a bowl.
2. Distribute the mixture into each lettuce leaf, as if you are filling a boat, and serve

Per Serving Calories: 516 Fat: 71g Carbohydrates: 3g Protein: 35g

19 - Tarragon Chicken Roast

Preparation	Cooking	Servings
15 min	**50 min**	**6**

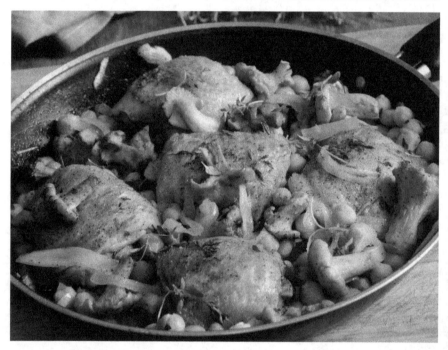

Ingredients

- 3 bone-in chicken thighs
- 3 tbsp of fresh tarragon leaves, chopped
- 3 shallots, thoroughly chopped
- 2 tbsp of garlic salt
- 3 tbsp of olive oil

Direction

1. Preheat the oven to 380F/180 C.

2. In a small bowl, combine the olive oil, garlic salt, and tarragon with the shallots.

3. Brush the mixture over the chicken pieces.

4. Bake in a greased baking dish for 40 minutes and switch on the broiler for the last five minutes to form a light crust.

5. Serve with salad or cauliflower rice

Per Serving Calories: 451 Fat: 34g Carbohydrates: 4.2g Protein: 34g

20 - Chicken Curry with Cauliflower Rice

Preparation	Cooking	Servings
15 min	15 min	6

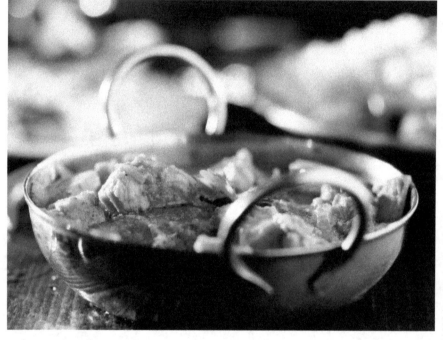

Ingredients

- 2 lb chicken (6 breasts)
- 2 packet curry paste
- 4 tbsp ghee (can substitute with butter)
- 1 cup heavy cream
- 2 head cauliflower (around 1 kg/2.2 lb)

Direction

1. Melt the ghee in a pot. Mix in the curry paste.

2. Add the water and simmer for 5 minutes.
3. Add the chicken, cover, and simmer on medium heat for 20 minutes or until the chicken is cooked.
4. Shred the cauliflower florets in a food processor to resemble rice.
5. Once the chicken is cooked, uncover, and incorporate the cream.
6. Cook for 7 minutes and serve over the cauliflower.

Per Serving Calories: 252 Fat: 17.2g Carbohydrates: 5g Protein: 14g

21 - Delicious Chicken Blanket

Preparation	Cooking	Servings
15 min	**45 min**	**6**

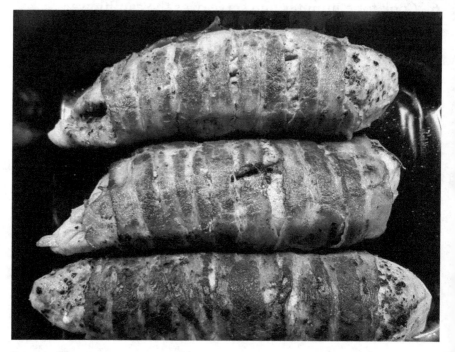

Ingredients

- 6 boneless chicken breasts
- 2 package beef bacon
- 1 8-oz package cream cheese
- 4 jalapeno peppers
- Salt, pepper, garlic powder, or other seasonings

Direction

1. Cut the chicken breast in half lengthwise to create two pieces.
2. Cut the jalapenos in half lengthwise and remove the seeds.
3. Dress each breast with a half-inch slice of cream cheese and half a slice of jalapeno. Sprinkle with garlic powder, salt, and pepper.
4. Roll the chicken and wrap 2 to 3 pieces of bacon around it—secure with toothpicks.
5. Bake in a preheated 375°F/190°C oven for 50 minutes.
6. Serve!

Per Serving Calories: 370 Fat: 28g Carbohydrates: 3.2g Protein: 1.8g

FISH

22 - Mesmerizing Shrimp Scampi

Preparation	Cooking	Servings
30 min	120 min	8

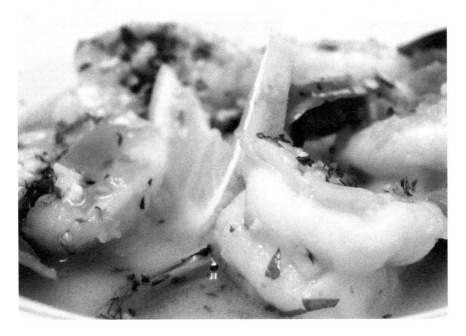

Ingredients

- 2 cup chicken broth
- 1 cup white wine vinegar
- 3 tablespoons olive oil
- 3 teaspoon garlic, chopped
- 3 teaspoons garlic, minced
- 2 pound large raw shrimp

Direction

1. Add chicken broth, lemon juice, white wine vinegar, olive oil, lemon juice, chopped garlic, and fresh minced parsley

2. Add thawed shrimp (the ratio should be 1 pound of shrimp for ¼ cup of chicken broth)

3. Place lid and cook on LOW for 2 and a ½ hours

4. Serve and enjoy!

Per Serving Calories: 283 Fat: 23g Carbohydrates: 3g Protein: 15g

23 - Sea Bass Spicy Hazelnuts

Preparation	Cooking	Servings
15 min	20 min	6

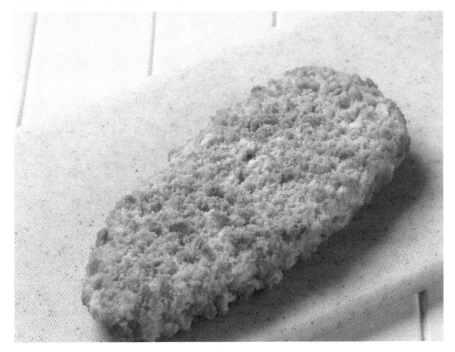

Ingredients

- 6 sea bass fillets
- 3 tbsp butter
- 1/2 cup roasted hazelnuts
- A pinch of cayenne pepper

Direction

1. Preheat your oven to 425⁵F.

2. Line a baking dish with waxed paper. Melt the butter and brush it over the fish.
3. Process the cayenne pepper and hazelnuts in a food processor to achieve a smooth consistency. Coat the sea bass with the hazelnut mixture.
4. Place in the oven and bake for about 15 minutes

Per Serving Calories: 417 Fat: 24g Carbohydrates: 2.8g Protein: 2.3g

24 - Grilled Salmon Marinated

Preparation	Cooking	Servings
45 min	15 min	6

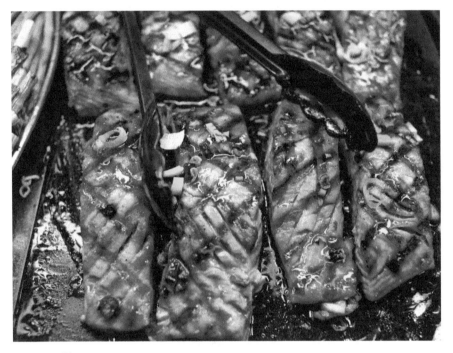

Ingredients

- 5-ounce salmon steaks
- 3 cloves garlic, pressed
- 6 tablespoons olive oil
- 1 tablespoon Taco seasoning mix
- 4 tablespoons fresh lemon juice

Direction

1. Place all of the above ingredients in a ceramic dish; cover and let it marinate for 40 minutes in your refrigerator.
2. Place the salmon steaks onto a lightly oiled grill pan; place under the grill for 6 minutes.
3. Turn them over and cook for a further 5 to 6 minutes, basting with the reserved marinade; remove from the grill.
4. Serve immediately and enjoy

Per Serving Calories: 312 Fat: 3g Carbohydrates: 25g Protein: 1.4g

25 - Salmon Fat Balls

Preparation	Cooking	Servings
20 min	**0 min**	**6**

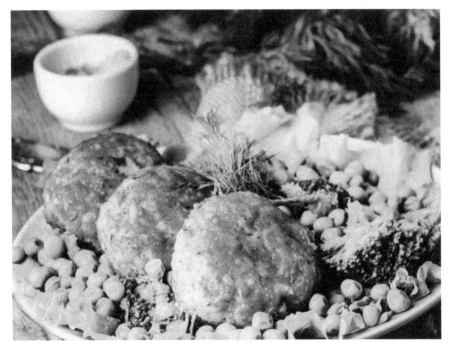

Ingredients

- 3 tbsp cream cheese, softened
- 2 ounce smoked salmon
- 3 tsp bagel seasoning

Direction

1. Take a medium bowl, place cream cheese and salmon in it, and stir until well combined.

2. Shape the mixture into balls, roll them into bagel seasoning and then serve

Per Serving Calories: 44 Fat: 5g Carbohydrates: 0.6g Protein: 2.5g

SOUPS

26 - Broccoli Soup and Cheese

Preparation	Cooking	Servings
15 min	40 min	6

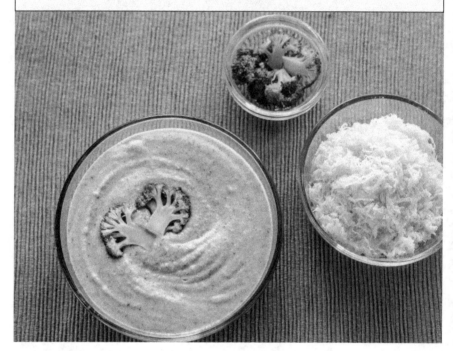

Ingredients

- 24 ounces chicken broth
- 15-ounce Velveeta low-fat cheese
- 3 bag frozen broccoli
- 14-ounce tomatoes and green chili pepper

Direction

1. Add frozen broccoli, tomatoes, broth, and chili to a pot.

2. Mix them well and place the pot over medium heat.

3. Bring it to a boil.

4. Then reduce the heat and simmer for 25 minutes.

5. Add cubed Velveeta into the soup.

6. Simmer until the cheese melts.

7. Serve hot and enjoy!

Per Serving Calories: 142 Fat: 4.2g Carbohydrates: 10.4g Protein: 8g

27 - Chicken Liver Stew

Preparation	Cooking	Servings
15 min	25 min	6

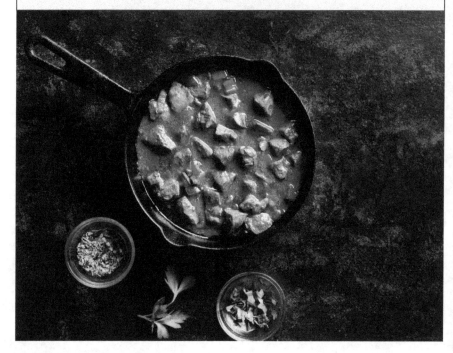

Ingredients

- 15 ounces chicken livers
- 3 ounces sour cream
- Salt, to taste
- 1-ounce onion, chopped
- 2 tablespoon olive oil

Direction

1. Place a pan over medium heat.

2. Add oil and let it heat up.

3. Add onions and fry until it turns brown.

4. Put livers and season with salt.

5. Cook till the livers become half-cooked.

6. Take a stew pot and transfer the mix.

7. Add sour cream and cook for 20 minutes.

8. Serve hot and enjoy!

Per Serving Calories: 129 Fat: 9.1g Carbohydrates: 2.3g Protein: 14g

28 - Chicken and Mushroom Stew

Preparation	Cooking	Servings
15 min	40 min	8

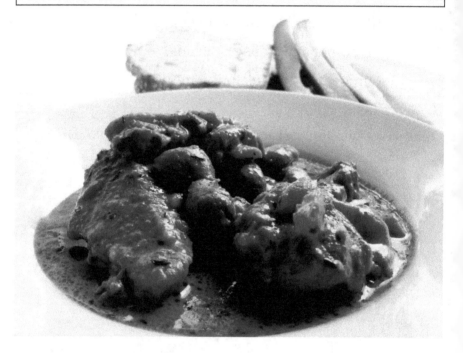

Ingredients

- 8 chicken breast halves, cut into bite-sized pieces
- 8 tablespoons olive oil
- 2 teaspoon thyme
- 2-pound mushrooms, sliced (5-6 cups)
- 2 bunch spring onion, chopped

Direction

1. Take a large deep-frying pan and place it over medium-high heat.

2. Add oil into it and let it heat up.

3. Put chicken and cook for 4-5 minutes for each side.

4. Add spring mushrooms and onions, season with salt and pepper as you need.

5. Stir it well, and then cover the lid.

6. Bring the mix to a boil.

7. Reduce the heat and simmer for 25 minutes.

8. Serve and enjoy!

Per Serving Calories: 217 Fat: 12g Carbohydrates: 11g Protein: 22g

29 - Garlic Chicken Soup

Preparation	Cooking	Servings
15 min	10 min	6

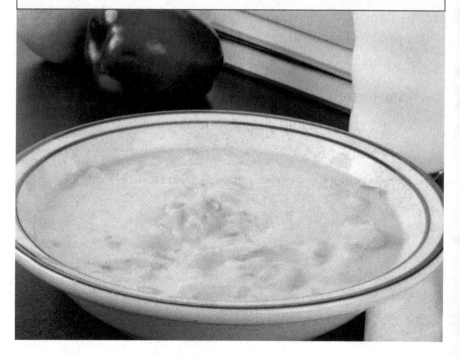

Ingredients

- 3 tablespoons butter
- 6 ounces cream cheese, cubed
- 18.5-ounce chicken broth
- 3 cups chicken, shredded
- ¼ cup heavy cream
- 2 tablespoons Stacey Hawkins Garlic Gusto Seasoning

- Salt, to taste

Direction

1. Take a saucepan and place it over medium heat.
2. Add butter into the saucepan and melt the butter.
3. Put the shredded chicken to the pan and coat with melted butter.
4. Add cream cheese and Stacey Hawkins garlic gusto seasoning when chicken is warm.
5. Mix to blend the ingredients.
6. Add chicken broth, heavy cream, and evenly distributed cream cheese.
7. Bring them to boil, then reduce the heat to low.
8. Simmer for 3-4 minutes.
9. Add salt to taste and serve.
10. Enjoy!

Per Serving Calories: 317 Fat: 21g Carbohydrates: 2.1g Protein: 11g

DESSERTS

30 - Bacon and Chocolate

Preparation	Cooking	Servings
25 min	25 min	8

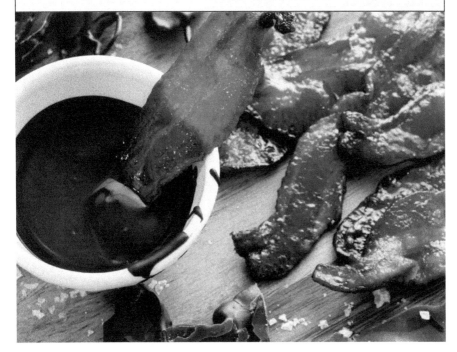

Ingredients

- 16 beef bacon slices
- 6 tablespoons unsweetened dark chocolate
- 2 tablespoons coconut oil
- 3 teaspoons liquid stevia

Direction

1. Preheat your oven to 425 degrees F
2. Skewer bacon into iron skewers

3. Arrange skewers on a baking sheet and bake for 15 minutes until they show a crispy texture

4. Transfer to a cooling rack

5. Take a saucepan and place it over low heat, add coconut oil and let it melt

6. Stir in coconut chocolate and heat until it melts

7. Add stevia and gently stir

8. Place crispy bacon on parchment paper and drizzle chocolate mix

9. Let the chocolate harden

10. Serve!

Per Serving Calories: 228 Fat: 24g Carbohydrates: 2.5g Protein: 6g

31 - Berries Yogurt Popsicles

Preparation	Cooking	Servings
5 hours	**0 min**	**8**

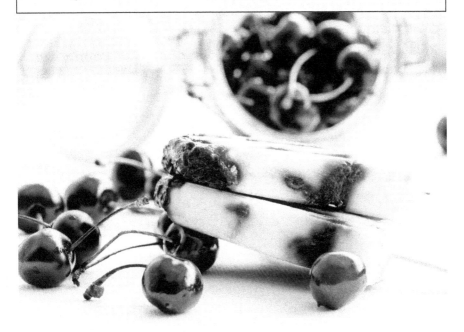

Ingredients

- 14 ounces frozen mango, diced

- 14 ounces frozen strawberries

- 2 cup Greek yogurt

- 5 teaspoons heavy whip cream

- 2 teaspoon vanilla essence

Direction

1. Blend the listed ingredients into your blender.

2. Blend until smooth.

3. Pour the mix into Popsicle molds.

4. Keep in the fridge for 3-5 hours.

5. Serve and enjoy!

Per Serving Calories: 187 Fat: 21g Carbohydrates: 8.2g Protein: 4.3g

32 - Lemonade Fat Bomb

Preparation	Cooking	Servings
20 min	0 min	4

Ingredients

- 2 whole lemon
- 8 oz of cream cheese
- 4 oz of butter
- 4 tsp of natural sweetener

Direction

1. Take a fine grater and zest your lemon

2. Squeeze lemon juice into a bowl alongside the zest
3. Add butter, cream cheese to a bowl and add zest, salt, sweetener, and juice
4. Stir well using a hand mixer until smooth
5. Spoon mix into molds and let it freeze for 2 hours
6. Serve and enjoy!

Per Serving Calories: 304 Fat: 41g Carbohydrates: 5.2g Protein: 4.1g

33 - Choco Fat Bombs

Preparation	Cooking	Servings
80 min	0 min	8

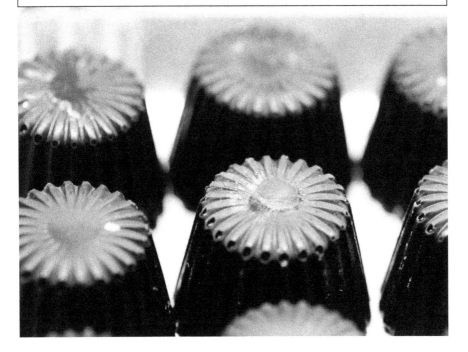

Ingredients

- 1 c of coconut oil

- 1 c of cocoa butter

- 20 drops vanilla-flavored stevia drops

Direction

1. Take a small saucepan and place it over medium heat
2. Add coconut oil and butter, let it heat up until combined
3. Remove heat and stir in stevia until combined well

4. Pour mix into muffin tins and transfer to freezer

5. Let it chill for 1 hour

6. Serve and enjoy!

Per Serving Calories: 327 Fat: 20g Carbohydrates: 4.2g Protein: 10g

34 - Vanilla Spiced Fat Bomb

Preparation	Cooking	Servings
90 min	**0 min**	**8**

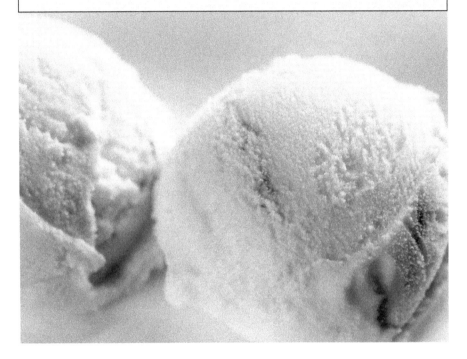

Ingredients

- 1 c of pumpkin puree

- 1 c of hemp seeds

- 1 c of coconut oil

- 4 tsp of pumpkin pie spice

- 2 tsp of vanilla extract

Direction

1. Take a blender and add all of the ingredients
2. Blend them well and portion the mixture out into silicon molds
3. Allow them to chill and enjoy!

Per Serving Calories: 113 Fat: 11g Carbohydrates: 4.2g Protein: 1.5g

35 - Raspberry Chocolate Cups

Preparation	Cooking	Servings
70 min	0 min	8

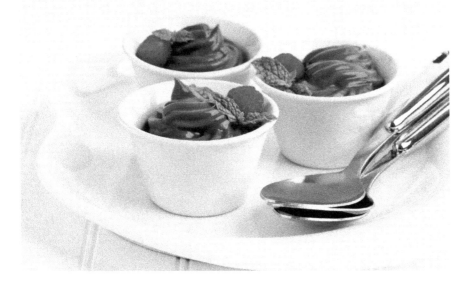

Ingredients

- ½ c of cacao butter and coconut manna
- 4 tbsp of powdered coconut milk
- 3 tbsp of granulated stevia
- 1 tsp of vanilla extract
- ¼ c of dried and crushed raspberries, frozen

Direction

1. Prepare your double boiler to medium heat and melt cacao butter and coconut manna
2. Stir in vanilla extract
3. Take another dish and add coconut powder and sugar substitute
4. Stir the coconut mix into the cacao butter, 1 tablespoon at a time, making sure to keep mixing after each addition
5. Add the crushed dried raspberries
6. Mix well and portion it out into muffin tins
7. Chill for 60 minutes and enjoy!

Per Serving Calories: 148 Fat: 14g Carbohydrates: 2g Protein: 2.8g

36 - Cold Coconut Bombs

Preparation	Cooking	Servings
2 hours	**0 min**	**8**

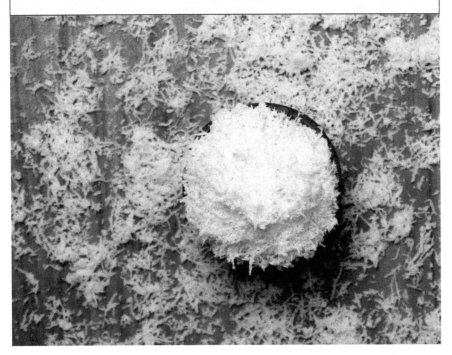

Ingredients

- 20 ounces coconut milk

- 1 c of coconut oil

- 2 c of unsweetened coconut flakes

- 30 drops of stevia

Direction

1. Microwave your coconut oil for 20 seconds in the microwave

2. Mix in coconut milk and stevia in the hot oil

3. Stir in coconut flakes and pour the mixture into molds

4. Let it chill for 60 minutes in the fridge

5. Serve and enjoy!

Per Serving Calories: 133 Fat: 12g Carbohydrates: 2.1g Protein: 1.3g

37 - Almond Butter and Coco Bomb

Preparation	Cooking	Servings
30 min	0 min	8

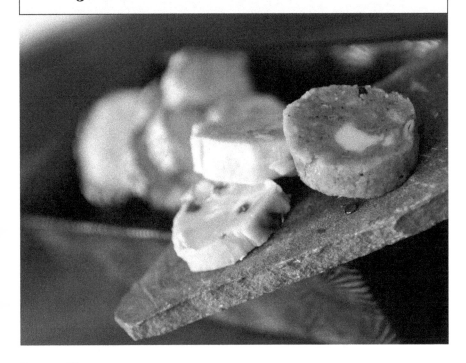

Ingredients

- 1/2 c of melted coconut oil
- 16 and ½ tbsp of almond butter + 9 tbsp salted butter
- 100 drops of liquid stevia
- tbsp cocoa

Direction

1 Take a bowl and add all of the listed ingredients

2   Mix them well
3   Pour scant 2 tablespoons of the mixture into as many muffin molds as you like
4   Chill for 20 minutes and pop them out
5   Serve and enjoy!

Per Serving Calories: 135 Fat: 13g Carbohydrates: 2g Protein: 1.5g

VEGAN AND VEGETARIAN

38 - Hearty Brussels Salad

Preparation	Cooking	Servings
10 min	15 min	4

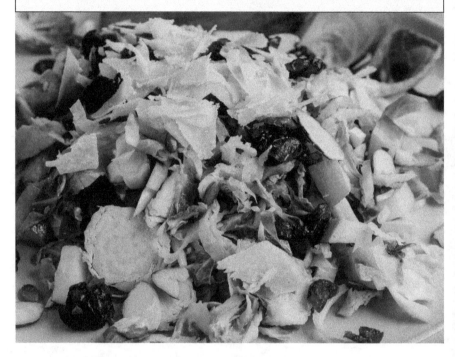

Ingredients

- 1 cup parmesan cheese, grated
- 1 cup hazelnuts, whole and skinless
- 2 tablespoon olive oil
- 2 pound Brussels sprouts
- Salt to taste

Direction

1. Pre-heat your oven 350-degree F
2. Line a baking sheet with parchment paper and trim bottom of Brussels
3. Put leaves in a medium sized bowl, making sure that they are broken
4. Toss leaves with olive oil and season with salt
5. Spread leaves on baking sheet
6. Roast for 10-15 minutes until crispy
7. Divide between bowls and toss with remaining ingredients
8. Serve and enjoy!

Per Serving Calories: 277 Fat: 18g Carbohydrates: 12g Protein: 13g

39 - Caramelized Onion

Preparation	Cooking	Servings
20 min	9 hours	8

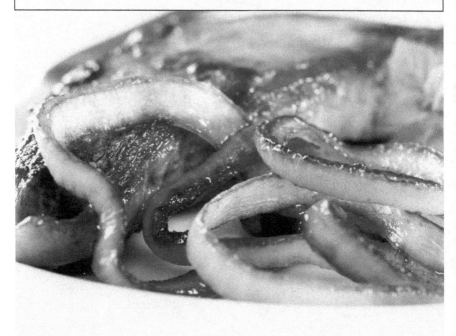

Ingredients

- 12 onions, sliced
- 4 tablespoons oil
- 1 teaspoon salt

Direction

1. Add onions, oil, and salt to your Slow Cooker.
2. Close lid and cook on LOW for 8 hours.

3. Open the lid and keep simmering for 1-2 hours until any excess water has evaporated.

4. Serve and enjoy!

Tip: If you don't have a slow cooker, you may use an Iron-Cast Dutch Oven. The temperature is 200 Degrees F for LOW and 250 degrees F for HIGH

Per Serving Calories: 116 Fat: 14g Carbohydrates: 14g Protein: 3g

40 - Broccoli Crunch

Preparation	Cooking	Servings
20 min	3 hours	8

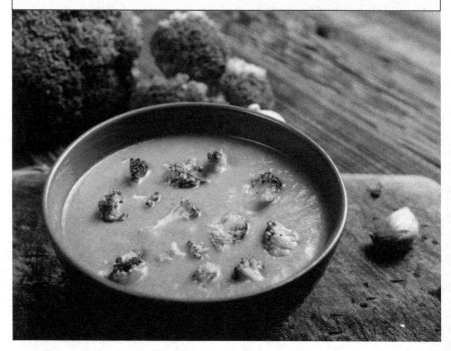

Ingredients

- 4 cups broccoli florets + 1 small yellow onion, chopped
- 4 ounces cream of celery soup
- 4 tablespoons cheddar cheese, shredded
- ¼ teaspoon Worcestershire sauce
- 1 tablespoon butter

Direction

1. Add broccoli, cream, cheese, onion, cheddar to Slow Cooker

2. Stir and season with salt and pepper

3. Place lid and cook on LOW for 3 hours

4. Serve and enjoy!

Tip: If you don't have a slow cooker, you may use an Iron-Cast Dutch Oven. The temperature is 200 Degrees F for LOW and 250 degrees F for HIGH

Per Serving Calories: 152 Fat: 10g Carbohydrates: 10g Protein: 5.2g

41 - Slow Cooked Brussels

Preparation	Cooking	Servings
25 min	**4 hours**	**8**

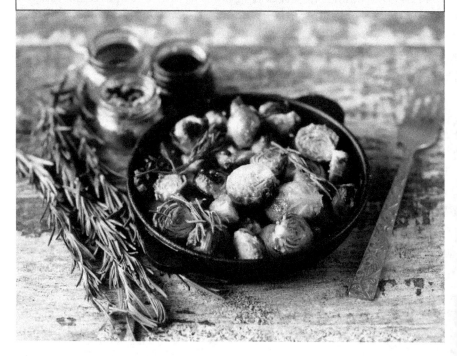

Ingredients

- 4 pound Brussels sprouts, bottom trimmed and cut
- 4 tablespoon olive oil
- 4 tablespoon Dijon mustard
- 2 cup water
- 2 teaspoon dried tarragon

Direction

1. Add Brussels, salt, water, pepper, mustard to Slow Cooker

2. Add dried tarragon and stir

3. Place lid and cook on LOW for 5 hours until the Brussels are tender

4. Stir well and add Dijon over Brussels

5. Stir and enjoy!

Tip: If you don't have a slow cooker, you may use an Iron-Cast Dutch Oven. The temperature is 200 Degrees F for LOW and 250 degrees F for HIGH

Per Serving Calories: 73 Fat: 4.2g Carbohydrates: 10g Protein: 4.1g

42 - Mixture Green Bean

Preparation	Cooking	Servings
15 min	2 hours	4

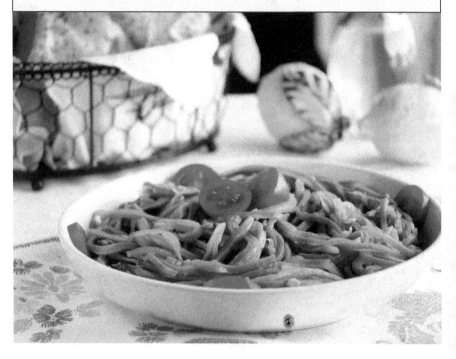

Ingredients

- 8 cups green beans, trimmed
- 4 tablespoons butter, melted
- 2 tablespoon date paste
- Salt and pepper as needed
- 1 cup slice tomato
- 1 teaspoon coconut aminos

Direction

1. Add green beans, date paste, pepper, salt, coconut aminos, and stir
2. Toss and place lid
3. Cook on LOW for 2 hours
4. Serve and enjoy!

Per Serving Calories: 216 Fat: 5g Carbohydrates: 7g Protein: 5g

43 - Leeks Platter Creamy

Preparation	Cooking	Servings
15 min	30 min	8

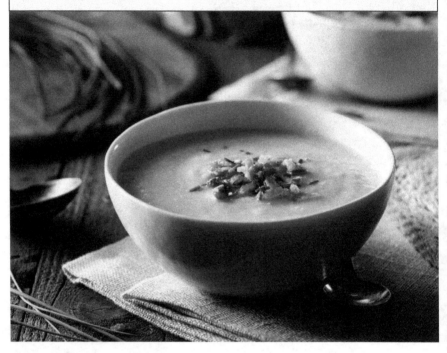

Ingredients

- 3 pound leeks, trimmed and chopped into 4-inch pieces
- 4 ounces butter
- 2 cup coconut cream
- 5 and ½ ounces cheddar cheese
- Salt and pepper to taste

Direction

1. Preheat your oven to 400 degrees F

2.   Take a skillet and place it over medium heat, add butter and let it heat up

3.   Add leeks and Saute for 5 minutes

4.   Spread leeks in greased baking dish

5.   Boil cream in a saucepan and lower heat to low

6.   Stir in cheese, salt, and pepper

7.   Pour sauce over leeks

8.   Bake for 15-20 minutes and serve warm

9.   Enjoy!

Per Serving Calories: 214 Fat: 14g Carbohydrates: 8g Protein: 6g

44 - Cheesy Cauliflowers

Preparation	Cooking	Servings
15 min	25 min	8

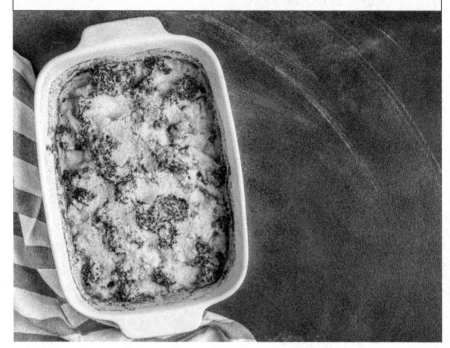

Ingredients

- 2 cauliflower head
- 1 cup butter, cut into small pieces
- 2 teaspoon Keto-Friendly Mayo
- 2 tablespoon Keto-Friendly Mustard
- 1 cup parmesan cheese, grated

Direction

1. Preheat your oven to 390 degrees F

2. Add mayo and mustard in a bowl
3. Add cauliflower to mayo mix and toss
4. Spread cauliflower in a baking dish and top with butter
5. Sprinkle cheese on top
6. Bake for 25 minutes
7. Serve and enjoy!

Per Serving Calories: 218 Fat: 21g Carbohydrates: 6.2g Protein: 3.1g

REFRESHING DRINKS AND SMOOTHIES

45 - Green Energizer Smoothie

Preparation	Cooking	Servings
15 min	**0 min**	**4**

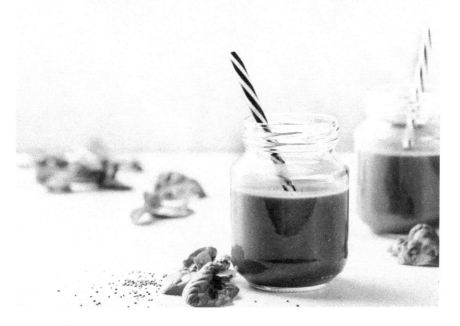

Ingredients

- 1 ripe mango, pitted and sliced
- 2 cup kale, chopped
- 6 cups baby spinach
- 2 cup of coconut water

Directions

1. Add all the ingredients except vegetables/fruits first
2. Blend until smooth
3. Add the vegetable/fruits

4. Blend until smooth
5. Add a few ice cubes and serve the smoothie
6. Enjoy!

Per serving Calories: 200 Fat: 12g Carbohydrates: 14g Protein: 8g

46 - Pineapple and Carrot Smoothie

Preparation	Cooking	Servings
15 min	0 min	4

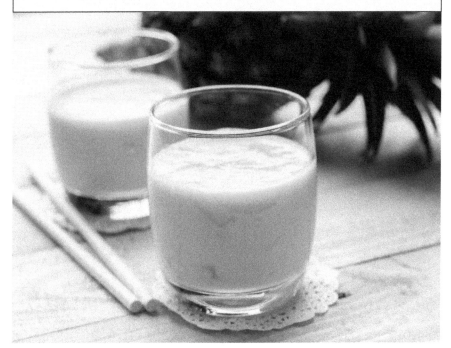

Ingredients

- 1 teaspoon cinnamon
- 2 cup fresh pineapple
- 6 organic carrots, scrubbed and sliced
- 10 cups baby spinach
- 2 large cucumber, diced

Directions

1. Add all the ingredients except vegetables/fruits first
2. Blend until smooth

3. Add the vegetable/fruits
4. Blend until smooth
5. Add a few ice cubes and serve the smoothie
6. Enjoy!

Per serving Calories: 92 Fat: 0.5g Carbohydrates: 14g Protein: 1.2g

47 - Mango Smoothie Energizer

Preparation	Cooking	Servings
15 min	0 min	4

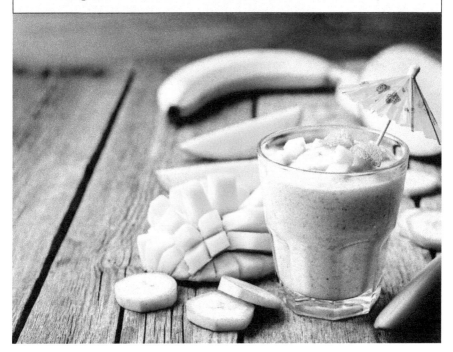

Ingredients

- 8 tablespoon protein powder
- 4 teaspoons spirulina
- 2 teaspoon bee pollen
- 2 frozen banana, sliced
- 2 cup of frozen mango, sliced
- 2 cups baby spinach
- 2 cup unsweetened almond milk

Directions

1. Add all the ingredients except vegetables/fruits first
2. Blend until smooth
3. Add the vegetable/fruits
4. Blend until smooth
5. Add a few ice cubes and serve the smoothie
6. Enjoy!

Per serving Calories: 146 Fat: 2.2g Carbohydrates: 18g Protein: 5.2g

48 - Green Frenzy Smoothie

Preparation	Cooking	Servings
15 min	0 min	4

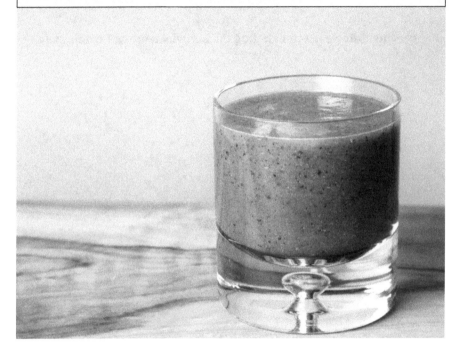

Ingredients

- 2 cup ice
- 4 tablespoons almond butter
- 2 teaspoon spirulina
- 6 teaspoon fresh ginger
- 3 frozen bananas, sliced
- 4 cups baby spinach, chopped
- 2 cup kale
- 3 cups unsweetened almond milk

Directions

1. Add all the ingredients except vegetables/fruits first
2. Blend until smooth
3. Add the vegetable/fruits
4. Blend until smooth
5. Add a few ice cubes and serve the smoothie
6. Enjoy!

Per serving Calories: 250 Fat: 4.2g Carbohydrates: 14g Protein: 24g

49 - Evergreen Morning Smoothie

Preparation	Cooking	Servings
15 min	0 min	4

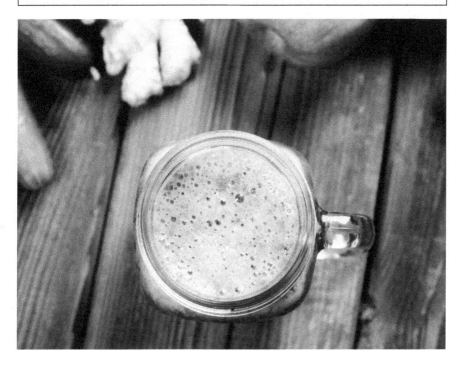

Ingredients

- 1 cup ice
- 2 cup kale, chopped
- 2 large red bell pepper, diced
- 2 large kiwi, peeled
- 2 scoop collagen protein powder
- Pinch of cayenne
- 1 lemon, juice

- 1 cup of water

Directions

1. Add all the ingredients except vegetables/fruits first
2. Blend until smooth
3. Add the vegetable/fruits
4. Blend until smooth
5. Add a few ice cubes and serve the smoothie
6. Enjoy!

Per serving Calories: 147 Fat: 1.8g Carbohydrates: 14g Protein: 11g

50 - Freshly Berries Smoothie

Preparation	Cooking	Servings
10 min	0 min	4

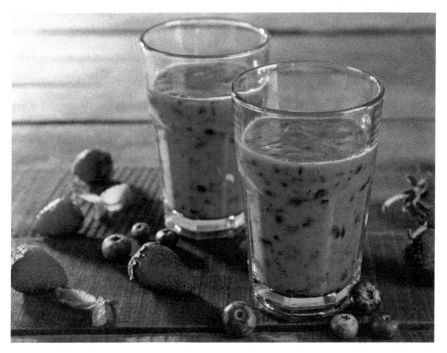

Ingredients

- 2 cup frozen blueberries
- 1 cup red bell pepper, chopped
- 1 cup seeded cucumber, diced
- 2 cup collard greens, chopped
- 6 stalks celery, chopped
- 1 teaspoon fresh ginger, peeled and minced
- 1 cup fresh flat-leaf parsley, chopped
- 2 scoop collagen protein powder

- 2 tablespoon freshly squeezed lemon juice
- 2 tablespoon freshly squeezed lime juice
- 1 cup of water

Directions

1. Add all the ingredients except vegetables/fruits first
2. Blend until smooth
3. Add the vegetable/fruits
4. Blend until smooth
5. Add a few ice cubes and serve the smoothie
6. Enjoy!

Per serving Calories: 155 Fat: 1.4g Carbohydrates: 13g Protein: 11g

CPSIA information can be obtained
at www.ICGtesting.com
Printed in the USA
LVHW082314230521
688301LV00003B/100

9 781639 300020